Real Fitness for Real Life: Practical Steps to a Healthier You

By
John Primrose

"Here, fitness meets practicality, ensuring your path to health fits your way of life."

Published by Real4Real Books
2024

Real Fitness for Real Life: Practical Steps to a Healthier You

Table of Contents

I'm Glad You're Here!

First and foremost, thank you for choosing my book and welcome to your first step toward a happier, healthier you! My name is John Primrose, and with over a decade of dedication to health and fitness, I've navigated the highs and lows of my own fitness journey. This book is the culmination of all that hard-earned knowledge. It's designed to be a realistic, accessible guide for people of all lifestyles and body sizes, emphasizing that everyone can achieve wellness. Whether you're just beginning or seeking to elevate your current routine, this guide is equipped with the insights, inspiration, and techniques necessary for success. Let's embark on this transformative journey together, unlocking the potential for a healthier, more vibrant you. Here, fitness meets practicality, ensuring your path to health fits your way of life.

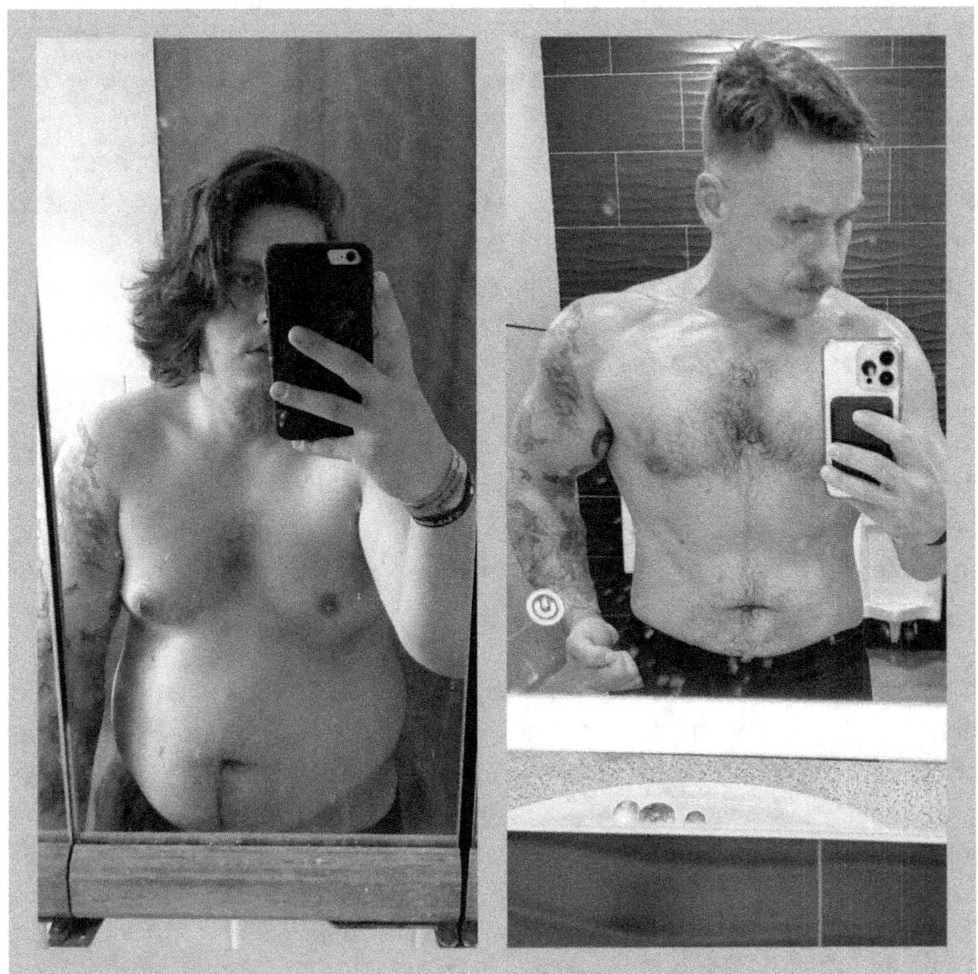

What You Can Expect

In "Real Fitness for Real Life," you're about to embark on a comprehensive fitness journey tailored to all levels of experience. Here's a preview of what this guide offers:

Techniques: Dive into a variety of exercise techniques suitable for different stages of your fitness journey. Starting with foundational exercises like squats, push-ups, and lunges, you'll learn the correct forms to ensure safety and effectiveness. As you progress, you'll explore intermediate strategies such as interval training and compound movements, before advancing to sophisticated methods like periodization and using supersets. Each technique is broken down with clear, step-by-step instructions.

Tips: Enhance your routine with valuable insights on nutrition, recovery, and mindset. From the importance of a balanced diet and hydration to the crucial roles of flexibility and rest in recovery, these tips are crafted to help you avoid common obstacles and sustain your motivation. You'll learn how to adapt your eating habits to support your energy needs and discover recovery techniques that prepare you for sustained success.

Plans: Uncover detailed workout plans that evolve with your fitness level. Begin with simple routines that build a strong base, then transition through more challenging intermediate workouts that increase in intensity and complexity. Finally, tackle advanced workouts that integrate unique equipment and demanding exercises for peak performance. Each plan is carefully structured to progressively challenge your body and drive positive results.

By the end of "Real Fitness for Real Life," you won't just understand the mechanics of achieving and maintaining a great physique—you'll be equipped with the knowledge, skills, and confidence to thrive in your new fitness lifestyle. Let's start this transformative journey together and unlock the best version of yourself!

Chapter 1: Understanding Fitness Fundamentals

Why Knowing How Your Body Works Can Help

When you start getting into fitness, it's really helpful to know a bit about how your body functions. Think of your body as a machine with different systems that help you move, breathe, and do activities. Here's a simple breakdown:

- **Muscles:** These are like the engine that powers your movements. When you exercise, you're basically training your muscles to be stronger and more efficient. Some exercises help you sprint fast or jump high (power), while others let you keep going for a long time without getting too tired (endurance).

- **Heart and Blood Vessels:** This system is like your body's delivery service. It pumps blood, which carries oxygen and nutrients to your muscles and carries away waste products like carbon dioxide. Activities like jogging, biking, or swimming make this system stronger and more efficient, which is great for your overall stamina and health.

- **Bones:** Think of your bones as the framework that holds everything together. Keeping your bones strong is crucial, and you can do this through activities that make you move your own body weight or lift weights.

Understanding these basics can help you choose exercises that focus on safety and enhancing the benefits of your specific fitness journey.

Remember, every small step you take towards understanding your body brings you closer to achieving your fitness goals. Embrace this knowledge and let it guide you towards a healthier, stronger you.

Exercise Is Really Good for You, Who Would've Thought?

Exercising regularly is one of the best things you can do for your health, and its benefits go way beyond just how you look:

- **Preventing Illness:** Staying active can help keep serious diseases like diabetes and heart disease at bay, and even help you maintain a healthy weight.

- **Boosting Your Mood:** Ever notice how you feel better after a workout? That's because exercise releases chemicals in your brain that make you feel happier and more relaxed.

- **Better Sleep:** Regular activity can help you fall asleep faster and sleep more deeply, as long as you don't exercise too close to bedtime.

- **More Energy:** Regular exercise strengthens your muscles and improves your endurance, which means you can do more without getting tired.

Exercise Musts: Because Your Body Will Thank You Later

To get the most out of exercising, I recommend mixing in different types of workouts:

- **Strength Training:** This type involves using weights or your own body weight to build muscle. It's not just about bulking up; stronger muscles and tissues make everyday activities easier and keep your bones healthy.

- **Cardio:** Any exercise that gets your heart rate up fits into this category. It's great for burning calories and keeping your heart healthy. Walking, running, and biking are all good cardio activities.

- **Flexibility Exercises:** These help keep your joints and muscles limber, which can prevent injuries and help you move better. Stretching and yoga are good examples.

Incorporating a little of each type of training into your routine is a great way to ensure a balanced approach to your fitness journey, helping you stay healthy and enjoy the things you love.

For me personally, being stronger, having better endurance, and being more flexible has helped me be a better dad. Playing with my boys is much more enjoyable now—mainly because I'm not the one begging for a timeout. And for that, I couldn't be more grateful.

Chapter 2: Setting Goals and Staying Motivated

Starting Fitness Goals Without Losing Your Sanity

Setting goals is like creating a personal roadmap for your fitness journey. To get started, you first need to understand where you're at right now. Think about what you can do comfortably today—maybe you can walk a mile without feeling too tired, or maybe you can do a few yoga poses. From there, you can start setting targets that are clear and reachable.

For example, if you currently walk a mile easily, you might set a goal to walk or run a 5K (which is about 3.1 miles) in three months. Or, if you're new to exercise classes, aim to attend three classes per week to get in the groove. Make sure your goals have a deadline and are specific enough that you'll know exactly when you've achieved them. This makes it easier to see your progress and stay focused.

How to Help Stay Motivated (Even When You'd Rather Nap)

Motivation is the spark that starts your fitness journey and the fuel that keeps it going. Here's how you can keep that motivation burning bright:

- **Set Small, Achievable Milestones:** Break your big goals into smaller ones. This could be as simple as improving your walking time each week or adding one more push-up to your routine every few days.

- **Celebrate Your Successes:** Give yourself a pat on the back every time you reach a milestone. Whether it's treating yourself to a movie or just doing a happy dance, celebrating makes you feel good and pushes you to continue.

- **Mix It Up:** Doing the same routine every day can get boring. Try different activities to keep your exercise exciting. If you usually walk, try a dance class. If you lift weights, mix in some swimming or sports.

This not only keeps you interested but also challenges different muscles.

- **Turning Motivation into Discipline:** Motivation is what gets you started, but discipline is what will keep you going long after the initial excitement fades. As you keep setting small goals, celebrating wins, and mixing things up, you're building habits that will turn fitness from a spark of motivation into a steady routine. Over time, showing up for yourself will become second nature, even on those days when you'd rather be napping. Remember, motivation may get you moving, but discipline will make sure you keep growing. Stick with it, and you'll find that what once felt like effort will soon feel like a natural part of your day. Keep pushing, and let discipline lead the way to lasting success!

Monitoring Your Milestones (Without the Stress)

Keeping an eye on your progress is not just motivating, it's also a crucial part of reaching your goals. Here are some simple ways to track your fitness journey:

- **Use a Fitness App:** There are many apps available that can help you monitor your activities, food intake, and more. These apps often offer tips and encouragement and make it easy to see how far you've come.

    - There are many fitness apps available that cater to different aspects of exercise and wellness. Here are a few popular ones that can help you track your fitness progress, set goals, and stay motivated:

    1. MyFitnessPal - This app is primarily known for its comprehensive food diary and calorie counter, but it also allows you to log your workouts and track your steps. It's great for monitoring your diet alongside your physical activity.

2. Strava - Popular among runners and cyclists, Strava tracks your runs and rides via your smartphone or GPS device. It provides detailed analytics on your performance and allows you to connect with friends and compete in challenges.

3. Fitbit App - Even without a Fitbit device, you can use the Fitbit app to track your daily steps, log activities, and record your workouts. If you do have a Fitbit, it syncs seamlessly with the device for detailed health and fitness monitoring.

4. Nike Training Club - This app offers a wide range of workout routines from strength to yoga, tailored to different fitness levels and durations. It features detailed instructions and videos to guide you through each exercise.

5. Zwift - Ideal for indoor cycling and running, Zwift combines the intensity of training with the fun of gaming. You can cycle or run in virtual environments while competing with other users from around the world in real-time.

6. YogaGlo - Perfect for those who want to practice yoga, this app provides access to thousands of yoga classes of varying styles and levels. You can pick classes based on duration, style, or specific teacher.

- **Keep a Fitness Journal:** If you prefer something more tangible, a fitness journal works great. Write down what you do each day, how long you did it, and how you felt afterwards. Over time, you'll have a clear picture of your progress.

- **Share on Social Media:** Sometimes, sharing your goals and progress with friends or on social media can offer an extra layer of support and accountability. Plus, you'll likely get encouragement from others, which can boost your motivation.

By using these strategies, you can not only set realistic and motivating goals but also enjoy every step of your fitness journey. Whether you're just starting out or have been at it for a while, remembering why you started and recognizing your progress can help you keep moving forward. Stay committed to your goals, and celebrate every milestone along the way. Your journey to fitness is a testament to your discipline, dedication and resilience. Keep pushing forward with confidence!

Chapter 3: Nutrition Basics for Fitness

Food and Fitness: The Dynamic Duo

Remember, think of your body like a machine (or a car) just as a car needs the right fuel to run well, your body needs the right food to perform at its best, especially when you're active. Fueling your body with the right foods empowers you to excel in your workouts and recover effectively, setting you on the path to achieving your fitness goals with renewed energy and vitality.

Basic Nutritional Guidelines for Energy and Recovery

Here's a simple way to think about what to eat to support your fitness activities:

- **Carbohydrates (Carbs):** These are your body's main energy source. Before a workout, carbs are like putting gas in the tank. Good sources include:

  - Simple Carbohydrates: Quick energy sources like fruit, honey, and even rice krispy treats (no food is bad if you understand its use and eat in moderation). They're fast to digest and can give you a quick energy boost which means they're ideal for 20-40 minutes before a workout. I normally eat my pre workout snack during my ten minute pre workout walk.

  - Complex Carbohydrates: These include whole grains, legumes, and starchy vegetables like potatoes. They take longer to digest, providing a more sustained energy release which is ideal for longer workout sessions, typically good to eat around 1-2 hours before your workout.

- **Proteins:** Think of protein as the repair kit for your muscles. After you exercise, protein helps repair and build up the muscle tissues that get broken down during a workout. You can find protein in foods like:

- Animal Proteins: These are complete proteins and include meat, fish, eggs, and dairy products. They contain all the essential amino acids your body needs.

- Plant-Based Proteins: These are found in foods like beans, lentils, tofu, and some grains like quinoa. Plant proteins are generally lower in one or more essential amino acids but can be combined with other plant sources to make a complete protein.

- **Fats:** While fats are often seen as something to avoid, they're actually essential for good health and provide a long-lasting energy source. Opt for healthy fats found in:

  - Unsaturated Fats: These are considered healthy fats and include options like olive oil, avocado, nuts, and seeds. They can help reduce inflammation and are good for heart health.

  - Saturated Fats: Typically found in animal products and some tropical oils. It's fine to have these in moderation, but they shouldn't be the main type of fat in your diet.

- **Hydration:** Drinking enough water is crucial, especially when you exercise, because you lose water through sweat. Staying hydrated helps you maintain your performance and recover better. Aim to drink water before, during, and after your workout.

Meal Prep Like a Pro (Or at Least Try)

Planning what you eat is just as important as planning a workout. Here are some tips to make meal planning simpler and more effective:

- **Include a Variety of Foods:** Each type of food gives you different nutrients. Try to include a colorful mix of foods in your meals—this usually means you're getting a good range of nutrients.

- **Prepare in Advance:** Life gets busy, and when you're tired or rushed, it's easy to grab whatever is quickest, often unhealthy options.

Preparing meals in advance can help you stick to healthy choices. Consider setting aside a few hours each week to prepare meals or at least a main protein source so that you have healthy options readily available.

- **Keep Healthy Snacks Handy:** Snacking isn't bad if you do it right. Keep healthy snacks like fruits, nuts, yogurt, or whole-grain crackers ready for when you get hungry. This helps prevent you from reaching for chips or sweets.

By focusing on good nutrition, you're not just eating better; you're also supporting your overall fitness goals, making every workout count, and improving your health and well-being. Whether you're just starting your fitness journey or looking to enhance your performance, what you eat makes a big difference.

Fuel your body with the right nutrition, and watch as your energy and performance soar. Every healthy choice you make is a step towards a vibrant, energized life. Keep nourishing yourself with purpose!

Chapter 4: Using Diet as a Tool to Reach Your Fitness Goals

No matter what diet you follow—be it low-carb, vegetarian, keto, or anything else—the fundamental principles of caloric intake play a crucial role in achieving your fitness goals. Whether you aim to lose weight, gain muscle, or maintain your current physique, understanding and managing your calorie intake is essential.

The Basics of Caloric Balance: Calories In, Calories Out, and Your Waistline's Secret Formula

Calorie Deficit for Weight Loss: To shed those extra pounds, you need to consume fewer calories than your body burns. This is known as a calorie deficit. When your body is in a calorie deficit, it turns to stored fat for energy, leading to weight loss. Even if you're following a specific diet, the core principle remains the same: you must burn more calories than you consume.

Calorie Surplus for Muscle Gain: Conversely, to put on weight and gain muscle mass, you need to consume more calories than your body burns, creating a calorie surplus. This provides your body with the necessary energy and nutrients to build new muscle tissue during resistance training. Regardless of the type of diet you choose, ensuring a calorie surplus is essential for effective weight gain or "bulking."

Understanding Macronutrients

While calorie intake dictates whether you gain or lose weight, the composition of those calories—macronutrients—determines how your body uses them. As discussed earlier, the three main macronutrients are:

- **Carbohydrates:** The primary source of energy for your body, especially important for high-intensity workouts. Think of these as your body's premium fuel—perfect for powering through those high-intensity workouts without running out of gas!

- **Proteins:** Essential for muscle repair and growth, helping to rebuild tissues that get broken down during exercise. These are like the construction crew for your muscles, coming in to repair and build up everything you break down during a workout.

- **Fats:** Important for energy storage, hormone production, and cell function. Healthy fats support overall health. Think of these as the long-term energy storage and maintenance crew, keeping everything running smoothly behind the scenes.

Balancing these macronutrients according to your goals (e.g., higher protein intake for muscle building) helps optimize your body composition.

The Role of Tracking: Making Every Bite Count, Literally

Personalized Nutrition: Tracking your calorie and macronutrient intake allows for a tailored diet that aligns with your specific fitness goals. It provides a clear picture of your eating habits and enables precise adjustments.

Improved Accountability: Keeping a record of your food intake helps you stay accountable and make healthier choices, reducing the likelihood of overeating or making poor dietary decisions.

Enhanced Performance and Recovery: Proper nutrition fuels your workouts and aids recovery, ensuring you have the energy to perform at your best and recover efficiently.

Practical Tips for Effective Tracking

1. **Set Clear Goals:** Determine whether your primary goal is weight loss, muscle gain, or maintenance. Your daily caloric and macronutrient needs will depend on this goal.

2. **Use Technology:** Let apps like "MyFitnessPal" do the heavy lifting of tracking your food—so you can focus on lifting actual weights! These tools offer extensive food databases and make logging your meals simple and accurate.

3. **Plan Your Meals:** Preparing meals in advance ensures you meet your nutritional goals and reduces the temptation to opt for unhealthy options. Think of meal prepping as setting your future self up for success—no more last-minute dives into the cookie jar!

4. **Be Consistent and Honest:** Track your intake every day, including weekends and special occasions. Accurate tracking provides a truthful picture of your diet. Track your intake every day, even when you're tempted by that weekend pizza. Your future self will thank you!

5. **Adjust as Needed:** Regularly review your progress and adjust your diet accordingly. If you're not seeing the desired results, tweak your macro ratios or calorie intake.

Understanding Macros and Calories: Macros Unmasked

In your fitness journey, understanding and managing your intake of macronutrients (macros) and calories is crucial. Macros are the nutrients that provide energy and are essential for various bodily functions. The three main types of macros are:

- **Carbohydrates:** Your body's primary source of energy. They are vital for fueling workouts and daily activities.

- **Proteins:** Essential for muscle repair and growth. They help rebuild tissues broken down during exercise.

- **Fats:** Important for energy storage, hormone production, and cell function. Healthy fats support overall health.

Calories measure the amount of energy provided by food. Managing your calorie intake helps achieve fitness goals, whether it's losing weight, gaining muscle, or maintaining your current physique. While calories determine whether you gain or lose weight, macros have a significant impact on your body composition—how much muscle and fat you have.

Benefits of Tracking Macros and Calories: It's Worth the Effort

1. **Personalized Nutrition:** By tracking your macros and calories, you can tailor your diet to your specific fitness goals. Whether you're looking to lose fat, gain muscle, or maintain your weight, understanding your nutritional intake allows for more precise adjustments.

2. **Improved Accountability:** Keeping a record of what you eat helps you stay accountable. It's easier to make healthy choices and avoid overindulging when you see a clear picture of your daily intake.

3. **Enhanced Performance:** Properly fueling your body with the right balance of macros ensures you have the energy to perform your best during workouts. It aids in recovery and supports overall health.

4. **Better Weight Management:** Tracking calories helps in creating a calorie deficit or surplus, depending on your goals. This practice is fundamental for effective weight management.

5. **Optimized Body Composition:** Monitoring your macro intake allows you to optimize your body composition. Consuming the right balance of proteins, fats, and carbohydrates helps build muscle, reduce body fat, and achieve a leaner, more toned physique.

Counting Macros and Calories Without Going Nuts

Step 1: Determine Your Goals First, establish your fitness goals. Are you aiming to lose weight, build muscle, or maintain your current weight? Your goal will dictate your daily calorie and macro needs.

Step 2: Calculate Your Needs I highly advise using an online calculator to determine your daily calorie and macro needs. One recommended website is "MyFitnessPal". This tool considers your age, gender, weight, height, and activity level to provide personalized recommendations. Here's how to get started:

1. Visit the "MyFitnessPal" website or download the app.

2. Create an account and enter your personal details.

3. Set your fitness goals (weight loss, muscle gain, maintenance).

4. Review the suggested daily calorie intake and macro distribution.

A common starting point for macros is:

- Carbohydrates: 45-65% of total calories

- Proteins: 20-35% of total calories

- Fats: 20-35% of total calories

Adjust these percentages based on your specific goals and dietary preferences.

Step 3: Track Your Intake Use a food diary or a tracking app like "MyFitnessPal" to log everything you eat and drink. These tools can break down your intake into macros and calories, making it easier to stay on track.

Step 4: Monitor and Adjust Regularly review your progress and adjust your intake as needed. If you're not seeing the desired results, tweak your macro ratios or calorie intake. Consistent monitoring helps you stay aligned with your goals.

Stay Sane and Track Smart: Practical Tips

- **Plan Your Meals:** Preparing meals in advance ensures you stick to your macro and calorie goals. It also reduces the temptation to opt for unhealthy options when you're hungry.

- **Stay Consistent:** Do your best to track your intake every day, even on weekends or during special occasions. Consistency is key to understanding your eating habits and making lasting changes.

- **Be Honest:** Record everything you consume, including small snacks, beverages, and even sauces (sauces can contain a lot of calories for a small amount of substance). Honesty in tracking provides an accurate picture of your diet.

- **Use Technology:** Take advantage of apps and devices that simplify tracking. Many apps have extensive databases of foods and can scan barcodes for easy logging.

- **Listen to Your Body:** While tracking is a valuable tool, also pay attention to how your body feels. Hunger, energy levels, and overall well-being are important indicators of whether your diet is working for you.

Tracking macros and calories might seem daunting at first, but with practice, it becomes a seamless part of your fitness routine. This method was a game-changer for me. It played a huge role in how I lost weight and transformed my body. By keeping track of exactly what I was eating, I could see how it impacted my progress (for better or for worse). This habit not only helped me reach my fitness goals but also completely changed the way I think about food and health. Don't stress, I promise you shouldn't have to do it forever (unless you want to). Over time, you should develop a solid understanding of the calorie content and macronutrient composition of the foods you enjoy eating. If you make tracking a part of your daily routine, you'll likely see major improvements in both how you look and feel.

Chapter 5: Workout Plans for Beginners

From Flop to Fit: Perfecting Basic Exercise Forms

Starting your fitness journey means getting to know a few key exercises that will form the foundation of your routine and help set you up for long term success. Here's how to do a few basic ones:

- **Squats:** Stand with your feet shoulder-width apart. Bend your knees and push your hips back as if you're sitting in a chair. Keep your back straight and your chest up. Squats work your thighs, hips, and buttocks.

- **Push-ups:** Start in a plank position with your hands under your shoulders. Lower your body until your chest nearly touches the floor, then push back up. Keep your body in a straight line from head to heels. Push-ups strengthen your chest, shoulders, and arms.

- **Lunges:** Step forward with one leg and lower your hips until both knees are bent at about a 90-degree angle. Make sure your front knee is directly above your ankle and your back knee doesn't touch the floor. Lunges target your legs and glutes.

Learning these exercises with the right form is crucial—it ensures you get the most out of the workout and significantly reduces the risk of injury.

Workout Plans for Rookies: Start Smart, Finish Strong

When you're new to exercise, the key is to start simple and slowly ramp up the intensity. Here's how to build a beginner-friendly workout plan:

- **Mix it Up:** A good workout plan includes a bit of everything. Aim to do strength training, cardio (like walking, cycling, or swimming), and flexibility exercises (like stretches or yoga) throughout the week.

- **Keep it Manageable:** Begin with exercises that are easy to perform and don't require complex movements or equipment. This helps build your confidence and strength without overwhelming you.

Sample 4-Week Beginner Program

Let's break down what a simple four-week plan could look like:

- **Week 1:** Focus on mastering the form of basic exercises. Use light weights or just your body weight. Keep cardio sessions short—think 10 to 15 minutes of brisk walking or any other low-intensity cardio you enjoy.

- **Week 2-4:** As you get more comfortable, start to challenge yourself a little more each week. Increase the weights slightly—if you're lifting, this might mean going from two pounds to five pounds. For cardio, slowly increase the duration. Start adding a few minutes each session until you're doing 20 to 30 minutes.

- **Stretch Regularly:** After every workout session, spend some time stretching. This helps in muscle recovery and flexibility. Basic stretches after working out can include things like reaching down to touch your toes, pulling your arm across your chest to stretch your shoulder, or gently pulling your heel to your buttock to stretch your thigh.

- **Keep Evolving:** As you finish this four-week plan, keep assessing your progress and adjusting your workouts. Maybe increase the weights, add more intervals, or try entirely new exercises. The goal is to keep challenging your body so you continue to improve.

The hope is to make your fitness journey less intimidating. By starting slowly, mastering the basics, and gradually increasing the difficulty, you'll set yourself up for success and make fitness a natural part of your daily routine. Every step you take in your fitness journey, no matter how small, is a victory. Believe in your potential and stay consistent. The foundation you're building today will lead to the strength and confidence you seek tomorrow. You'll soon find that incorporating exercise into your life is not only achievable but also enjoyable and rewarding.

Chapter 6: Intermediate Workout Strategies

Moving On Up: Goodbye Beginner, Hello Progress

With a solid foundation in place, it's time to elevate your workouts and push those boundaries, embracing new challenges with some new found confidence. Here's how to move from beginner to intermediate:

- **Add Weights:** If you've been doing bodyweight exercises, start incorporating weights. This can be anything from holding a dumbbell while doing squats to using a barbell for bench presses.

- **Try New Movements:** Explore exercises that challenge you in new ways. For example, if you've mastered the basic squat, try a one-legged squat or add a jump at the end of your squat.

Intermediate Fitness: More Sweat, More Fun

At the intermediate level, you can start introducing more complex workouts that push your fitness further:

- **Interval Training:** This involves alternating short bursts of intense activity with intervals of lighter activity. For example, after a 2-minute brisk walk, you could run at full speed for 30 seconds, then slow down and repeat.

- **Compound Movements:** These exercises work multiple muscle groups at once and are great for building overall strength and efficiency. Examples include bench presses, deadlifts, and weighted squats. These not only work your major muscles but also engage your smaller, stabilizing muscles.

Sample 4-Week Intermediate Program

Here's a simple plan to guide your transition to more challenging workouts:

- **Week 1:** Start adding weights to exercises you're already comfortable with. For instance, if you've been doing air squats, hold a dumbbell in each hand this week.

- **Week 2:** Introduce interval training into your cardio sessions. You could start with something straightforward like 1 minute of jogging followed by 1 minute of walking, and repeat.

- **Week 3:** Begin doing compound exercises. A good start might be doing a push-up into a side plank, combining upper body strength with core stabilization.

- **Week 4:** Start challenging yourself with more advanced variations of familiar exercises. If you're doing yoga, try poses that require more balance and strength, like Warrior III or Crow Pose.

Moving to an intermediate level is exciting because it allows you to push yourself more and see even greater improvements in your fitness and overall well-being. The key is to progress gradually and listen to your body to avoid overdoing it. Embrace the challenge, and you'll continue to grow stronger and more confident in your abilities. Your commitment to progress is a testament to your strength. Keep pushing your limits, and you'll find yourself achieving feats you once thought impossible.

Chapter 7: Advanced Training Techniques

For the Fitness Fanatic: Advanced Workouts

As your fitness journey progresses, it's time to integrate advanced training techniques that will push your limits and help you overcome plateaus, propelling you toward your peak performance Here's a look at some sophisticated strategies:

- **Periodization**: This is a fancy way of saying you vary your workout intensity and focus over time. It's like planning your year with phases of hard work and easier periods to help your body recover and grow stronger. You might spend a few weeks focusing on building strength, then switch to focusing on speed or endurance.

- **Supersets**: This technique involves doing two different exercises back-to-back with no rest in between. It's a great way to make your workouts more challenging and time-efficient. For example, you might do a set of push-ups immediately followed by a set of pull-ups.

- **Drop Sets**: This involves performing an exercise until failure, then reducing the weight and continuing for additional reps. This technique maximizes muscle fatigue and growth.

- **Pyramid Sets**: You increase the weight and decrease the reps with each set, then reverse the process. This strategy effectively builds strength and endurance.

- **Compound Sets**: Similar to supersets, but both exercises target the same muscle group, increasing the intensity and focus on that area.

Sample 4-Week Advanced Program

Here's how you might structure a four-week program using advanced techniques:

Week 1: Introduce Supersets: Pair exercises that target opposite muscle groups (like biceps and triceps) to keep the intensity high without overworking one area. For example, do a set of bicep curls immediately followed by tricep dips.

Week 2: Focus on Periodization: Increase the weight and lower the number of reps in your strength exercises to focus on power. For instance, if you've been doing 3 sets of 12 reps, try 4 sets of 6 reps with heavier weights.

Week 3: Incorporate Drop Sets: After completing your final set of an exercise, reduce the weight by about 20-30% and continue to lift until failure. For example, after completing 4 sets of bench press, immediately reduce the weight and continue to press until you can't lift anymore.

Week 4: Mix in Advanced Equipment Exercises: Use kettlebells for swings or resistance bands for added resistance in squats and presses. Combine these with Pyramid Sets for a full challenge. Start with a lower weight and higher reps, increase the weight while decreasing reps, then reverse.

Detailed Weekly Breakdown:

Week 1: Supersets

- Monday: Upper body (e.g., push-ups/pull-ups, bicep curls/tricep dips)

- Wednesday: Lower body (e.g., squats/hamstring curls, lunges/calf raises)

- Friday: Full body (e.g., deadlifts/rows, kettlebell swings/burpees)

Week 2: Periodization

- Monday: Strength (heavy weights, low reps: deadlifts, bench press, squats)

- Wednesday: Power (moderate weights, moderate reps: clean and press, box jumps)

- Friday: Endurance (light weights, high reps: circuit training, bodyweight exercises)

Week 3: Drop Sets

- Monday: Upper body (bench press, shoulder press, followed by drop sets)

- Wednesday: Lower body (leg press, leg extension, followed by drop sets)

- Friday: Full body (pull-ups, rows, followed by drop sets)

Week 4: Advanced Equipment and Pyramid Sets

- Monday: Kettlebell swings (pyramid sets), resistance band squats

- Wednesday: TRX rows (pyramid sets), medicine ball slams

- Friday: Battle ropes (pyramid sets), weighted vest lunges

Specialized Equipment: Toys for Serious Fitness Fans

Advanced equipment can introduce new challenges and stimulate your muscles in unique ways:

- **Stability Balls**: These are large inflatable balls used for various exercises. They're great for improving balance and core strength because you have to work to keep stable while performing exercises like crunches or planks.

- **TRX Bands (Suspension Trainers)**: These are tools that use gravity and your body weight to perform hundreds of exercises. You can adjust your body position to add or decrease resistance, making it a versatile piece of equipment for full-body workouts.

- **Kettlebells**: These cast-iron weights are great for dynamic exercises that combine strength, endurance, and flexibility. Exercises like kettlebell swings, goblet squats, and Turkish get-ups can provide a full-body workout.

- **Resistance Bands**: These flexible bands add resistance to exercises and are excellent for strength training, flexibility, and rehabilitation. They come in various tension levels and can be used for exercises like bicep curls, squats, and lateral band walks.

- **Foam Rollers**: These cylindrical tools are used for self-myofascial release, helping to relieve muscle tightness, soreness, and inflammation. They are great for post-workout recovery and improving flexibility.

- **Battle Ropes**: These heavy ropes are used for high-intensity workouts that improve cardiovascular endurance and strength. They are perfect for exercises like rope slams, waves, and alternating waves.

- **Medicine Balls**: These weighted balls are ideal for explosive strength training and functional fitness. They can be used for exercises like medicine ball slams, throws, and rotational twists.

- **Weighted Vests**: Adding extra weight with a vest can increase the intensity of bodyweight exercises like push-ups, pull-ups, and running. It helps build strength and endurance.

- **Plyometric Boxes**: These sturdy boxes are used for plyometric exercises that improve explosive power and agility. Exercises like box jumps, step-ups, and lateral box shuffles are great for enhancing athletic performance.

- **Ab Wheels**: This simple yet effective tool targets the core muscles, providing a challenging workout. Rolling the wheel out and back helps build abdominal strength and stability.

Using these advanced techniques and equipment can dramatically boost your strength, balance, and overall fitness. These methods are intense, so make sure you're ready for them and always prioritize proper form to avoid injuries.

As you complete this four-week plan, keep pushing yourself to evolve. Regularly assess your progress and adjust your workouts—whether it's increasing the weights, adding more intervals, or trying entirely new exercises. The key is to keep challenging your body to continue improving.

Remember, the beginner, intermediate, and advanced training techniques provided are guides and suggestions. Use them to find what fits best into your routine and personal fitness journey. Customize these strategies to match your goals, preferences, and lifestyle. Your fitness journey is unique, and it's all about discovering what works best for you.

Stay motivated and embrace the process of finding your rhythm. Celebrate every achievement, no matter how small. Keep evolving and growing stronger, one step at a time. Your discipline and dedication will lead to amazing results, and you'll be proud of how far you've come. Keep pushing forward, and enjoy every moment of your fitness journey!

Chapter 8: Flexibility and Recovery

Flexibility and Recovery: The Yin to Your Workout's Yang

While flexibility and recovery might not have the same excitement as intense workouts, they are vital components of any fitness routine, ensuring long-term success and well-being. They help prevent injuries by keeping your muscles and joints happy and healthy, and they give your body a chance to repair and grow stronger after your workouts.

- **Flexibility:** This refers to the ability of your muscles to stretch. The more flexible you are, the better your body can move during exercises and everyday activities, reducing the risk of getting hurt.

- **Recovery:** This is the time you give your body to heal and replenish energy after exercising. Proper recovery not only prevents injuries but also ensures you're ready to perform well in your next workout. Think of your recovery days as spa days for your muscles—they've earned it!

Flex Appeal: Stretching Routines for Everyone

Incorporating a daily stretching routine can significantly improve your flexibility and reduce muscle tightness and soreness. Here's how to get started:

- **Focus on Major Muscle Groups:** Include stretches for your legs, back, arms, and shoulders. Each stretch should be held gently without pain for about 20-30 seconds.

- **Consistency is Key:** Try to stretch every day, especially after workouts when your muscles are warm. This can help improve your overall flexibility over time.

- **Dynamic vs. Static Stretching:** Before workouts, focus on dynamic stretches, which involve moving parts of your body and gradually increasing reach, speed, or both. After workouts, use static stretches, where you hold a single position for a stretch without moving.

Reboot Your Body: Simple Recovery Techniques

Effective recovery involves several techniques:

- **Adequate Sleep:** Sleep is when most of your body's healing and growth occur. Aim for 7-9 hours of quality sleep per night to help your body recover from workouts.

- **Proper Nutrition:** Eating the right foods after you exercise can help replenish your energy stores and repair muscle tissues. Focus on a mix of proteins for muscle repair and carbohydrates to refill energy.

- **Active Recovery:** This involves doing light, non-strenuous activities on your rest days, like walking, gentle yoga, or easy swimming. These activities help increase circulation and aid the recovery process without straining your muscles.

- **Hydration:** Drinking enough water is essential for recovery. It helps flush out toxins, transports nutrients to your cells, and keeps your muscles functioning properly.

Sauna Secrets: Why Sweating Feels So Good

To get the most benefit from sauna use, spend about 15-20 minutes in the sauna after your workout. Ensure you stay hydrated by drinking plenty of water before and after your sauna session. Always listen to your body and exit the sauna if you feel dizzy or uncomfortable. Effective recovery involves several techniques:

- **Muscle Relaxation**: The heat from the sauna helps relax muscles and relieve tension, making it an excellent post-workout recovery tool.

- **Improved Circulation**: The heat causes blood vessels to dilate, which increases blood flow and improves circulation. This enhanced circulation can help speed up muscle recovery and reduce soreness.

- **Detoxification**: Sweating in the sauna helps flush out toxins from the body. This detoxification process can contribute to overall health and well-being.

- **Stress Relief**: Saunas provide a calming environment that can help reduce stress and promote mental relaxation. The heat stimulates the release of endorphins, which are natural mood enhancers.

- **Enhanced Immune Function**: Regular sauna use can boost the immune system by increasing the production of white blood cells, which help fight off infections.

- **Better Sleep**: The relaxation effects of the sauna can lead to improved sleep quality. A good night's sleep is crucial for effective recovery and overall health.

Chill Out: The Power of Cold Plunges

Cold plunges, or quick dips in cold water, may sound intense, but they offer powerful recovery benefits:

- **Reduces Muscle Soreness:** Cold water reduces inflammation, easing next-day soreness after intense workouts.

- **Speeds Recovery:** By helping flush out lactic acid, cold plunges can get you back to training sooner.

- **Boosts Circulation:** After a plunge, blood flow increases, delivering fresh oxygen and nutrients to muscles for quicker healing.

- **Mental Toughness:** Embracing the chill builds resilience, strengthening both body and mind.

How to Cold Plunge Safely:

1. **Start Slow:** Begin with 1-2 minutes in 50-59°F water, then gradually increase as you feel comfortable.

2. **Listen to Your Body:** Exit if you feel discomfort. Warm up slowly afterward to avoid sudden temperature shifts.

Incorporating techniques like stretching, proper nutrition, adequate sleep, active recovery, sauna and cold plunge use can significantly enhance your recovery process and overall well-being. By focusing on flexibility and recovery, you're not just helping your body mend—it's also a crucial step in preparing yourself for more challenging workouts in the future. This approach ensures that your fitness journey is sustainable and enjoyable, keeping you healthy and active for a long time.

Chapter 9: Overcoming Plateaus and Keeping Fit Long Term

Stuck in a Rut? Understanding Fitness Plateaus

Hitting a fitness plateau, where progress stalls despite ongoing effort, is common. This often occurs because your body adapts to your routine or workout intensity, signaling it might be time for some new challenges. Here are some common reasons why plateaus occur:

- **Repetitive Routines:** Doing the same exercises with the same intensity every day can lead your body to hit a comfort zone, where it no longer feels challenged.

- **Insufficient Intensity:** If your workouts don't challenge you enough, your body might not have a reason to improve further.

Level Up: Strategies to Conquer Fitness Plateaus

Breaking through a plateau means changing things up and giving your body a new challenge. Here's how you can do that:

- **Mix Up Your Routines:** Try different exercises or activities to keep things interesting and challenging. If you usually run, try cycling or a dance class.

- **Increase Intensity:** Boost the difficulty level of your workouts by adding more weight, increasing speed, or doing more repetitions. This helps push your body out of its comfort zone.

- **Supportive Diet:** Make sure you're eating enough food and the right kind of food to fuel your workouts. Sometimes, a lack of progress can be due to not eating enough or not getting the right nutrients.

Lifelong Fitness: Tricks to Keep the Couch at Bay and Your Spirits High

Keeping fit for life isn't just about avoiding plateaus; it's about making fitness a sustainable part of your lifestyle. Here are some tips to help you stay fit in the long run:

- **Adopt Fitness as a Lifestyle:** Instead of viewing exercise as a chore, try to see it as a regular part of your life. This mindset helps you keep moving even when you don't feel like sticking to your routine.

- **Set New Goals:** Always have a new goal to aim for. Once you reach one goal, set another. This could be improving your time, lifting heavier weights, or preparing for a competitive event.

- **Try New Activities:** Keep your routine exciting by trying new sports or fitness classes. This not only helps prevent plateaus but also keeps you engaged and interested.

- **Join a Community:** Connect with others who share your fitness interests. Whether it's a local running club, a yoga class, or an online fitness community, being part of a group can provide motivation and support.

- **Consistency is Key:** Regular activity is more effective than intermittent intense workouts. Try to be consistent with your exercise, even if some days it's just a short walk.

By adopting these strategies, you can overcome the inevitable plateaus and keep your fitness journey exciting and rewarding for years to come. Fitness isn't just a short-term goal; it's a way to live a longer, healthier, and more fulfilling life. Embrace plateaus as opportunities to reassess and reignite your passion. Stay persistent, keep innovating, and your long-term commitment will lead to lasting transformation.

Recommended Reading and Resources for Fitness Enthusiasts

To enhance your fitness journey, consider utilizing these resources and incorporating the knowledge from these books to help you stay motivated and achieve your health and fitness goals more effectively.

Books:

- **"Starting Strength: Basic Barbell Training" by Mark Rippetoe** - This book is a comprehensive guide for beginners to advanced lifters focusing on the importance of strength training and proper technique.

- **"The 4-Hour Body" by Timothy Ferriss** - Ferriss offers methods for rapid body transformation, focusing on unconventional advice and 'body hacking' techniques.

- **"Becoming a Supple Leopard" by Kelly Starrett** - A must-read for anyone looking to improve mobility, resolve pain, and optimize athletic performance through detailed, illustrated guides on how to perform and modify movements to avoid and recover from injuries.

- **"You Are Your Own Gym" by Mark Lauren** - For those who prefer to train without weights, this book provides strategies for using bodyweight exercises to build strength at home.

- **"The Fitness Mindset" by Brian Keane** - Keane offers advice on how to eat for energy, train effectively, manage your mindset, and achieve long-term results.

Resources:

- **"MyFitnessPal"** - This app is an excellent tool for tracking your calorie and macro intake. It has an extensive database of foods, a barcode scanner for easy logging, and allows you to monitor your progress towards your fitness goals.

- **Strava** - Popular among runners and cyclists, Strava tracks your runs and rides via your smartphone or GPS device. It provides detailed analytics on your performance and allows you to connect with friends and compete in challenges.

- **Fitbit App** - Even without a Fitbit device, you can use the Fitbit app to track your daily steps, log activities, and record your workouts. If you do have a Fitbit, it syncs seamlessly with the device for detailed health and fitness monitoring.

- **Nike Training Club** - This app offers a wide range of workout routines from strength to yoga, tailored to different fitness levels and durations. It features detailed instructions and videos to guide you through each exercise.

- **Zwift** - Ideal for indoor cycling and running, Zwift combines the intensity of training with the fun of gaming. You can cycle or run in virtual environments while competing with other users from around the world in real-time.

- **YogaGlo** - Perfect for those who want to practice yoga, this app provides access to thousands of yoga classes of varying styles and levels. You can pick classes based on duration, style, or specific teacher.

Progress Tracking Template (Example)

Date	Weight	Body Fat %	Muscle Mass %	Notes
05/01/2024	180	20	40	Felt strong during workouts
05/08/2024	178	19.5	41	Increased cardio sessions
05/15/2024	177	19	41.5	Focused on high protein intake
05/22/2024	175	18.5	42	Added more veggies to diet
05/29/2024	174	18	42.5	Consistent with workouts

*To obtain body fat/muscle mass % I recommend purchasing a cheap digital scale that can calculate these percentages. You can find them on various online stores. Information in the chart is provided for example purposes only.

Workout Log Template (Example)

Date	Exercise	Sets	Reps	Weight	Notes
05/01/2024	Squats	3	12	100 lb	Focused on form
05/01/2024	Bench	3	10	80 lb	Increased weight by 5 lb
05/01/2024	Deadlift	3	8	120 lb	Felt strong

| 05/03/2024 | Pull-ups | 3 | 8 | Body | Need to improve grip strength |
| 05/03/2024 | Plank | 3 | 1 min | N/A | Held longer than last time |

Meal Plan Template (Example)

Day	Meal	Food Items	Cals	Protein	Carbs	Fats
Monday	Breakfast	Oatmeal, Banana, Almond butter	350	10g	50g	12g
Monday	Lunch	Grilled chicken salad	400	35g	30g	15g
Monday	Dinner	Burger, Air Fried Potatoes	620	45g	65g	20g
Monday	Snacks	Protein Shake	120	25g	2g	1g
Tuesday	Breakfast	Oatmeal, Banana, Almond butter	350	10g	50g	12g
Tuesday	Lunch	Grilled chicken salad	400	35g	30g	15g
Tuesday	Dinner	Burger, Air Fried Potatoes	620	45g	65g	20g
Tuesday	Snacks	Protein Shake	120	25g	2g	1g

*Calories are provided for example purposes only and may not be accurate. If you use this method of tracking, it's important to research the caloric content of your foods. I highly recommend using an app like 'MyFitnessPal' to track your nutrition accurately.

Conclusion: The Final Rep – Stronger Every Day

As we reach the end of our journey together, let's take a moment to celebrate the incredible strides you've made. This book has equipped you with a solid foundation to transform your fitness journey into a sustainable lifestyle. From mastering the essential techniques for building strength, cardio fitness, and flexibility to understanding the pivotal role of nutrition, you now have the tools for lasting success.

Fitness is more than just a series of exercises; it's a holistic approach to enhancing your overall well-being. Every rep, every meal, and every effort contributes to building a healthier, more vibrant you. By embracing balanced workouts and mindful eating, you are not just shaping your physique but nurturing a lifestyle that promotes vitality and happiness.

Remember, fitness is a marathon, not a sprint. It's about making steady progress and celebrating every milestone along the way. Adapt your routines as needed, find joy in your achievements, and keep pushing towards your goals. Your determination and commitment are the driving forces that will lead you to your best self.

Thank you for allowing me to be part of your transformative journey. Here's to your continued health, strength, and happiness. Keep pushing forward, keep learning, and always strive to be the best version of yourself. Together, we can achieve greatness, one step at a time. A happier, healthier you is just around the corner, starting with your next rep, your next healthy meal, and your next day dedicated to your goals.

Believe in your potential, embrace the journey, and let every step you take be a testament to your strength and resilience. You have the power to transform your life, one rep, one meal, and one day at a time. Let's continue to grow stronger together!

Appendix and References

Glossary of Terms

- **Cardiovascular Training:** Exercise aimed at improving the heart and blood vessels' ability to absorb and transport oxygen efficiently.

- **Flexibility Training:** Exercises designed to enhance the range of motion in muscles and joints.

- **Hypertrophy:** The enlargement of an organ or tissue from the increase in size of its cells; in fitness, it specifically refers to muscle growth.

- **Interval Training:** A method that alternates between bursts of high-intensity activity and periods of low-intensity activity or rest.

- **Periodization:** The organized approach to training that involves progressively cycling various aspects of a workout program during a specific period.

- **Plank/Side Plank:** A core-strengthening exercise where you hold your body in a straight line, supporting your weight on your forearms and toes (plank) or on one forearm and the side of one foot (side plank). It engages the core, shoulders, and lower back.

- **Reps (Repetitions):** The number of times an exercise is executed in one set without stopping.

- **Sets:** Groups of repetitions performed consecutively, usually with rest in between.

- **Superset:** A combination of two exercises performed back-to-back with no rest in between.

- **To Failure:** Performing an exercise until you can no longer complete a full, correct repetition due to muscle fatigue.

- **Isometric Exercise:** Exercises in which muscles contract without changing length, such as holding a squat or plank position.

- **Compound Exercise:** Movements that work multiple muscle groups simultaneously, like squats or deadlifts.

- **Active Recovery:** Light physical activity during rest days, such as walking or gentle stretching, aimed at promoting circulation and recovery without strenuous effort.

Scientific References and Credits

Books:

- Rippetoe, Mark. "Starting Strength: Basic Barbell Training." The Aasgaard Company.

- Ferriss, Timothy. "The 4-Hour Body." Crown Archetype.

- Starrett, Kelly. "Becoming a Supple Leopard." Victory Belt Publishing.

- Lauren, Mark. "You Are Your Own Gym." Light Of New Orleans Publishing.

- Keane, Brian. "The Fitness Mindset." CreateSpace Independent Publishing Platform.

Articles and Websites:

- "20 Best Fitness Books for Beginners." BookAuthority. BookAuthority

- "The 6 Best Fitness Books for Beginners." Livestrong. Livestrong

- "72 Best Fitness Books." Read This Twice. Read This Twice

The resources listed have been crucial in providing the scientific backing and practical insights discussed throughout this book. For further reading and to deepen your understanding of the topics covered, please refer to the detailed works mentioned above.

www.ingramcontent.com/pod-product-compliance
Lightning Source LLC
Chambersburg PA
CBHW051715250726
48653CB00007B/3044